WORKBOOK

For

KEEP SHARP

Build A Better Brain at Any Age

SANJAY GUPTA, MD

Roger Press Publishers

ISBN: 978-1-954432-20-8

Copyright © 2021 by: Roger Press

All rights reserved. This book or any portion thereof may not be reproduced or used in any manner whatsoever without the express written permission of the publisher except for the use of brief quotations in a book review.

TABLE OF CONTENTS

ABOUT THE AUTHOR 6
INTRODUCTION 7
NOTHING BRAINY ABOUT IT 7
PART 1 14
THE BRAIN: MEET YOUR INNER BLACK BOX 14
CHAPTER 1: WHAT MAKES YOU "YOU" 15
CHAPTER 2: COGNITIVE DECLINE—REDEFINED 25
    DR. RUDY TANZI'S "ALZHEIMER'S IN A DISH" 31
    KINDS OF COGNITIVE DEFICITS 32
CHAPTER 3: 12 DESTRUCTIVE MYTHS AND THE 5 PILLARS THAT WILL BUILD YOU 36
    THE DIRTY DOZEN 36
    HOW TO KEEP A SHARP MIND 40
PART 2: THE BRAIN TRUST 43
HOW NOT TO LOSE YOUR MIND 43
CHAPTER 4: THE MIRACLE OF MOVEMENT 44
    THE PACE OF AGING 44
    SMARTER AND BIGGER BRAINS IN MINUTES OF MOVEMENT 46
    MOVING THROUGH EVOLUTION 47
    SHAPE YOUR BRAIN BY GETTING INTO SHAPE 48
    JUST AS YOU WOULD BRUSH YOUR TEETH 49
CHAPTER 5: THE POWER OF PURPOSE, LEARNING, ... 52
AND DISCOVERY 52
    KEEPING THE BRAIN PLASTIC 52
    THE BRAIN AND COGNITIVE RESERVE 53
    THE DEFINITION OF "COGNITIVELY STIMULATING" ACTIVITIES 55
    GETTING IN THE FLOW 56

CHAPTER 6: THE NEED FOR SLEEP AND RELAXATION 59
    SLEEP MEDICINE 60
    THE RINSE CYCLE 61
    THE TOP TEN SECRETS TO SLEEP 61
CHAPTER 7: FOOD FOR THOUGHT 66
WHAT'S GOOD FOR THE HEART IS GOOD FOR THE BRAIN 68
    MY GUIDE TO GOOD EATING 69
    The Gluten Debate 70
CHAPTER 8: CONNECTION FOR PROTECTION 74
    THE SECRET SAUCE TO A LONG, SHARP LIFE 75
TIPS TO HELP YOU STAY SOCIALLY ACTIVE 76
CHAPTER 9: PUTTING IT ALL TOGETHER 80
12 WEEKS TO *SHARPER* 80
    WEEKS 1 AND 2: DIVE INTO THE FIVE 81
        WEEKS 3 AND 4 83
        WEEKS 5 AND 6 83
        WEEKS 7 AND 8 84
        WEEKS 9 AND 10 84
        WEEK 11 85
        WEEK 12 85
PART 3: THE DIAGNOSIS 88
WHAT TO DO, HOW TO THRIVE 88
CHAPTER 10 88
DIAGNOSING AND TREATING AN AILING BRAIN 88
    BRINGING HOPE 89
    A POUND OF PREVENTION 90
    THE THREE STAGES OF ALZHEIMER'S DISEASE 90
    DEMENTIA IMITATORS 92

THE MEDICAL CHECKUP	93
SOME OF THE NATIONWIDE ORGANIZATIONS/PROGRAMS LOOKING INTO DEMENTIA:	94
CHAPTER 11: NAVIGATING THE PATH FORWARD	**96**
FINANCIALLY AND EMOTIONALLY, WITH A SPECIAL NOTE TO CAREGIVERS	**96**
IT TAKES A VILLAGE	96
BRACE YOURSELF	98
KEEP TALKING	100
DON'T FORGET YOURSELF: A NOTE FOR CAREGIVERS	100
CONCLUSION	**105**
THE BRIGHT FUTURE	**105**

ABOUT THE AUTHOR

Sanjay Gupta's first and most real love is the **"BRAIN."** He spent four years to get a medical degree and another seven years concluding his residency training to be a neurosurgeon; he has been that for over twenty years now. Dr. Gupta has won his place three times in a row as a New York Times bestselling author and is presently the **Chief Medical correspondent for CNN**. He has written and reported major health headlines and documentaries which have gone down in history for his bravery in his reporting style even in the face of battles, diseases, and natural disasters all over the world. Amongst the documentaries attributed to his in-depth investigations are "One Nation Under Stress" for HBO and his "Weed Series."

Sanjay Gupta has bagged multiple Emmy awards, Peabody awards, and DuPont awards. He traveled around the world seeking ancient cultures that have defied the natural boundaries of death to enable him to be well equipped to write his nonfiction books – "Chasing Life, Monday Mornings: A Novel, and Cheating Death." His journalism accolades are quite colossal, asides from being regarded as the most trusted reporter in the media industry. He has received various honorary degrees and humanitarian awards due to his care and excessive concern for those incapacitated by war and natural disasters.

He was honored by a prestigious business magazine – Forbes, as one of the ten most influential celebrities, and in 2019, he was elected into the National Academy of Medicine which is one of the higher honors in the medical field. Sanjay Gupta lives in Atlanta and is married to a beautiful wife named Rebecca and three lovely daughters.

Gupta is an associate chief of neurosurgery at Grady Memorial Hospital and an associate professor of neurosurgery at Emory University Hospital, and also functions as a diplomate of the American Board of Neurosurgery.

INTRODUCTION
NOTHING BRAINY ABOUT IT

Dr. Gupta never set out to become a doctor or more so – a brain surgeon, all he wanted was to become a writer. At the age of thirteen, he chose medicine shortly after his grandpa went down with a stroke. The author watched how his grandfather's verbal response deteriorated fast, as he became unable to speak or write, but perfectly understood when spoken to and could read easily.

These observations got him interested in studying how the brain functions. At this tender age of thirteen, Dr. Gupta began to spend more time at the hospital asking surgeons a lot of medical inclined questions, got his answers, and also began reading up many materials on medicine and the human body. The doctors returned his grandfather to good health, by opening his carotid artery that allowed the flow of blood to his brain and avoids further strokes in the nearest future.

The memory aspect of the brain became Dr. Gupta's core interest. It fascinated this young mind that our memories, which signifies who we are, are summarized to be invisible neurochemical signals among miniature areas of the brain. In the early 1990s, he enrolled in medical school, and orthodox wisdom taught that brain cells like neurons didn't have the enablement to regenerate, but Dr. Gupta was rather optimistic that our brain cells cannot stop growing as long as we keep having new thoughts, renewed experiences, intense memories, and novel learnings all through our lifetime. In 2000 when he was done with his training on neurosurgery, his findings backed up his earlier optimism that of a truth, the brain can birth new brain cells called neurogenesis and also increase its size. The revelation here is that we all hold the control system to our bodies. Our brains can become sharper, fitter, faster and better if we train them to be. The choices we make either enhances or deters the functionality of the brain the more.

The focus here is to grow new brain cells and make the old ones work efficiently, and not necessarily dishing out ways to increase the brain's IQ or intelligence. This piece is about the brains' ability to efficiently handle short-term and long-term assessments of the world and how resilient the brain is to handle tough life challenges that are enough to cripple a man.

Cognitive decline has altered all over the years. The history of record on dementia goes as far back as 1550 BCE, as Egyptian doctors described the disorder as Ebers Papyrus. In 1797, a French psychiatrist, Philippe Pinel gave this disorder a befitting name called – "Dementia" which is Latin; meaning out of one's mind. The aforementioned psychiatrist is known as the father of modern psychiatry due to his immense contribution to psychiatry. In the 19th century, Dementia was simply known as a specific loss of one's cognitive ability.

During this period a British Physician – Dr. James Cowles Prichard published his book "A Treatise on Insanity" in which he introduced the term "senile dementia." Senile means old, in this case, it refers to the insanity that shows in older people as memory loss is one of the predominant symptoms of dementia, thereby associating the word to old aged people.

For a very long time, the word dementia was seen as an insult and referred to as a curse. There was so much negativity surrounding the word, forgetting the fact that dementia is a collection of symptoms connected to poor judgment and memory loss.

Dementia is vaguer than specific; it can be a spectrum ranging from mild to severe. Some of the causes of dementia are highly alterable, but for the record, Alzheimer's disease and dementia are not the same things, even though they have been prevalently used interchangeably in time past and even in present times.

There is nothing to be scared about as it concerns memory. Memory loss is only a misguided fear; it is not preordained. Many desire to have an improved brain but are limited with the options to make this desire a reality (that's if it is even possible). Our brains are not black boxes that are untouchable and without the capacity to improve. The brain can be improved, refreshed, and modified for as long as we live.

"Keep Sharp" will help you design your own "sharp brain" program that can be ingrained easily into your daily life. It will clarify why the brain acts in certain ways and why it doesn't act in ways you had hoped it would. And then teach you how to inculcate certain habits into your routine to make it seamless.

Many medical experts have a lot of advice to offer as to what foods are best eaten, activities to imbibe into our daily routine or even the amount of sleep the body needs. Thus, the reason for many contradictory messages on the internet and even in hard copies on healthy living and what is best for all. In summary, this is like a master class on how to build the best version of the brain, become more productive, and aid you in becoming that better mother, father, daughter, son, etc....

Once the brain is functioning optimally, clean and smooth; then other parts of the body has no option to follow suit. Now you make quality decisions, enhanced resilience, and be more optimistic. To take care of your body; take care of your mind first. Many fear losing their minds than even death itself. If that is the motivation you brought on board, change it now. What should drive you is the knowledge that you can build a better brain at any given age.

Resilience is the answer to building a better brain. A brain that can stand in the face of enduring trauma, think uniquely, and starve brain-related illnesses to preserve cognitive memory for optimal performance. Open up your minds to learning ways to keep the brain sharper, healthy and the methods entailed to build a better brain as we age. It is a possibility; it is not a fallacy.

Before we go on quickly to talk more in-depth on the brain, below are self-assessment questions to help you know whether you are at risk for brain degeneration as collated by neurologists. If you can answer these questions honestly, you can know where you stand as regards your brain's health. Whatever the case may be, note that these risk factors are all modifiable; so don't be terrified, you will not receive a doomsday analysis anytime soon or in the future, it's only best to know. They are as follows;

1. At the moment, are you suffering from any brain-connected ailment, or have been diagnosed in the past with mild cognitive deficiency?
2. Do you stay away from strenuous exercises?
3. Are you the type to sit down for the better part of the day?
4. Would you say you are overweight or even obese?
5. Are you a female?
6. Do you have a history of being diagnosed with cardiovascular disease?
7. Do you have any metabolic disorders like insulin resistance, high blood pressure, high cholesterol, or diabetes?
8. In the past have you been diagnosed with an infection with the possibility of leading to chronic inflammation that can have neurological effects (e.g., syphilis, Lyme disease, herpes)?
9. Are you in the habit of taking some medications that can affect the health of the brain, such as antihistamines, antianxiety drugs, antidepressants, or blood pressure drugs, statins, proton pump inhibitors?

10. Has it ever been established that you had a concussion, leading from a brain injury or head trauma, whether from an accident or while playing an impact sport?
11. Are you a habitual smoker or it was in the past?
12. Do you have a history of depression?
13. Do you struggle with social engagement with others?
14. Did you further your education after high school or didn't even get to high school level of formal education.
15. What does your diet consist of mostly, is it high in fatty foods, processed foods, sugary, and low in vegetables, whole grains, fresh fruits, nuts, fish, and olive oil?
16. Do you live with chronic, unrelenting stress? (Constant stress and is difficult to cope with.)
17. Any history of alcohol abuse?
18. Are you suffering from any sleep disorder or experience poor sleep daily?
19. Do you have hearing loss?
20. Is your entire day void of cognitive challenges, such as learning something new or playing game(s) that involves a lot of thinking?
21. Is your job void of complexities, like working with people where you function as their mentor, supervisor dishing out instructions and persuading them to work?
22. Are you above sixty-five years old?
23. Is Alzheimer's disease patrimonial for you or has the diagnosis revealed that you carry the "Alzheimer's gene variant," APOE3 or APOE4, or both?

24. Are you currently taking care of dementia or Alzheimer's disease patient?

If by any chance you said yes to more than five of the questions above, there is every possibility your brain is on the verge of declining. And if you didn't answer yes to more than three of the questions listed above, then it's about time to optimize the health of your brain to perform better. The rest of this workbook will reveal how the above questions relate to your brain's health.

PART 1
THE BRAIN: MEET YOUR INNER BLACK BOX

The brain sends electrical signals that make sure we can stand on our feet, move around, breathe, blink, feel and even think. Scientists say that the brain is the most multifaceted thing ever discovered, and the innovators of DNA say the brain is the last and magnificent biological frontier. The information in the brain moves through billions of neurons and it travels faster than the speed of a race car in motion.

How our brain function is the understanding behind who we are and how we experience the world. The brain shapes us, all we stand for, our connection with other humans, what brings us joy, what marvels us, even till when we rely totally on the brain to make tough but good decisions on our behalf, plan, and get us ready for what the future might hold.

The brain helps us to form memories, tells us stories in form of dreams when we are asleep, helps us adapt to different environments, and even tells time. We can call the brain the reservoir of our consciousness.

The brain is very demanding as it consumes 20% of the sum of blood and oxygen produced in the body even though it consists of approximately 2.5% of our body weight. The brain gives life.

CHAPTER 1: WHAT MAKES YOU "YOU"

The brain holds a larger part of what we are, what we will become, and how we define our world.

Many have tried to imagine what the brain looks like and visualize it as a dull and bland gray mass on the exterior. This is what the brain looks like – Pink with whitish-yellow coverings and big blood vessels flowing on and through it.

With deep fissures separating the brain into different lobes, called *sulci*, and mountainous peaks, recognized as *gyri*.

In an operation, the brain throbs softly on the borders of the skull and appears alive. The brain is a mystical and fragile organ that carries out a great deal of work despite its versatility and outstanding function. Likening the brain's ability to a computer is a terrible understatement for a body organ that weighs a little over three pounds. Our contemporary laptop computers weigh far more than the brain and the brain can perform in ways the computer can never compete. Is it in processing speed, storage capacity, motherboard, encodings, and encryptions? The brain outweighs any computer capacity and more.

The ways we perceive the world is influenced by the brain. Of a truth, the brain sees things upside down and the retina at the back of the eye sees images two-dimensionally from each eye, but the brain converts what is seen to three-dimensional images with great perception and a clear and rational image.

No matter how advanced and erudite artificial intelligence gets, there remain several things our brain can do that computers can't attempt. The human brain is about 1/40 of our body weight compared to that of an elephant which is 1/550 of their total weight.

The amazing ability of humans set us apart from other species even though all animals do their everyday business of sleeping, eating, reproducing, and enduring involuntary visceral processes regulated by the "reptilian brain". Our primitive reptilian brain influences our behavior greatly and our complex outer cerebral cortex (*Cortex* got from Latin meaning bark in Latin, just as the outer layer of the brain) helps us to carry out sophisticated duties such as creating tools, learning different languages, acquiring intricate skills and residing in a social group. The outer layer of the brain folds over and over into itself thereby making the surface area extremely larger than imagined.

The human brain encloses a projection of 100 billion brain cells and billions of more nerve fibers. The neurons in the brain are linked to tons of networks called *synapses*. These connections help us to think abstractly, remember things, feel angry, feel hungry, make decisive decisions, rationalize, use languages, be creative, think about the past, make plans towards the future, communicate our intentions, have moral standings, pass judgment, find solutions to complex problems, take note of scents in the air, sense fear or danger, tell lies or jokes, be angry, analyze information, and interpret emotions.

Every part of the brain has designated obligations that are linked together in a synchronized manner. The severe brain injury of Phineas Gage that made him the most famous survivor of an extreme brain injury, threw light into the revelation of the inner intricacies of the brain for many scientists which were expedient in a time when cutting-edge techniques weren't available to analyze the brain components discovered.

This twenty-five-year-old; Phineas Gage was greatly injured in 1848 while working at Cavendish, Vermont; on the construction of a railroad when a long iron rod lodged into his cheek penetrating his face, blinding his eye, going through his head, brain, and out to the top due to an explosive powder that detonated. Gage survived that injury, but his personality couldn't escape that traumatic event. He turned from a gentleman into a violent and undependable person. That was the first time a clear-cut link was created between trauma and specific regions of the brain as regards a personality change. Unfortunately, Gage died twelve years after the accident; but strange was recorded during the latter part of his life before his departure due to several seizures he encountered.

The mystifying occurrence referred to above was the taking place of *neuroplasticity*. This is reconnection and networking of areas in the damaged parts of the brain. In Gage's place, his brain began to show signs of healing and rehabilitation from his past trauma. The human brain is not static; it evolves as each day passes. It learns, grows, and mutates.

Though Gage's traumatic experience revealed how complex the human brain can be and its inevitable connection to our behavior; it is also important that we know that the magnificent power of the brain isn't attributed only to specific anatomical compartments but the communication and circuitry amid the sections that make up our complex feedbacks and behaviors.

In our thoughts about the brain, we wonder and ponder on the elements that make us "US". We brood over the mind and that voice that speaks to us all through the day. This inner voice controls your actions, gestures, raises vital and frivolous questions, makes decisions for us, makes us feel jealous, scared, and insecure, creates joy, hope, and pleasure inside of us, and even beats you up emotionally on several occasions.

In all the years of studying the brain, we are still yet to discover where our consciousness (being aware of oneself and his/her immediate surroundings) lives inside the brain, that is if it resides in the brain at all. What is definite is the part of the brain that is responsible for solving mathematical problems, learning new languages, networks responsible for processing sight, walking, planning, and many more. What no one can tell is precisely where your self-awareness streams from; there is a high possibility it is from a convergence of factors in the brain.

The brain holds no sensory fiber. No get to the brain, you have to cut open the skin to get to the skull and then the brain. The skin has pain fibers but the latter previously mentioned is void of its sensory receptors. That's why it is an option to perform brain surgery on a conscious patient. The brain is so delicate and vulnerable that too much pressure on some parts of the brain during a surgical operation can make or maim the individual for life.

Another way the brain is fragile and vulnerable is that it cannot be replicated/replaced in the advent of an extreme brain injury. Unlike the heart, kidney, and all. The brain has been put under lots of tests, close observation, and monitoring, and to date, scientists are yet to discover what makes it beat and what makes it slow down its pulse. This uncertainty has affected the comprehension and treating of neurodegenerative degeneration, complex disease progressions, and disorders of the brain, from autism to Alzheimer's.

With the site where our consciousness resides which is still in the vague, we as unique humans are well aware that we have a brain that is the powerhouse of the entire body, even though we cannot touch and feel it like we would to our skin, we do know it exists. That is a foremost pillar to aid a sharp, fast, and resilient brain.

THE ESSENCE OF MEMORY, THINKING, AND HIGH MENTAL FUNCTIONING

Memory is said to be "the mother of all wisdom" as said by the ancient Greek dramatist – Aeschylus. It is equally the mother of all we are about. Our various memories are what form our present experiences and give us a sense of self and identity in life. Memories give us a reason to live and make us feel capable and valued. Memories remind us of the past and make a connection along the decision-making lines in other to guide our future endeavors.

Memory is a very common cognitive function and the foundation of all learning because it is in it that we can store knowledge and process it as well. Our memory has the prerogative to decide the information worth storing and where it will be stored. Memory is not the same as memorizing. This is so because memory is not a warehouse for storing knowledge when not in use. It is wrong to liken memory to a physical building, memory is flexible and it changes constantly with the entrance of novel information.

Many of us, however, mistake memory for "memorizing." We view memory as a warehouse where we keep our knowledge when we are not using it, but that metaphor is not correct because memory is not static like a physical building. Our memories are constantly changing as we take in fresh information and interpret it. Our memory has to assist in building and maintaining an organized life following who we are as new experiences come in to cause changes in that regard.

The content of the memory is constantly being updated and changed. New information either adds up to preexisting related information or takes the position of the former and becomes the main go-to on that subject matter. Either way, our memory is constantly being modified. So we can say that our memories are not accurate and objective records of past events. Our memory is continually deducing and examining inbound information.

It is of utmost importance to remain cognitively intact all through our time on earth in other not to be patients of dementia and to achieve great feats in our professional careers. The construction of memory is to reconvene diverse memory images or impressions of cells found all over the brain. Simply put, our memory is not an isolated system but it consists of a network of systems that works in synchrony with specific roles to either create, store or recall events.

To improve and preserve memory at the cognitive level, you have to work on all functions of your brain. Memory hacks and tricks can be helpful but only in reinforcing some components of memory. Memory building occurs in the following stages –

- Encoding - it starts with the opinion of an experience with the use of your senses.
- Storage - this refers to short-term and long-term memory, alcohol for instance hinders the process of information moving from the short-term memory to the long-term memory section. It is during sleep that the transfer of events from the short-term memory to the long-term memory occurs. Some neurons in the body are responsible for letting the brain intentionally forget and it is actively functional during sleep. Our head is cleared of events that have stayed for a long time to create space for new information.

- Retrieval – this refers to calling up a memory. It starts from taking the recalled information from your unconsciousness to your conscious mind.

No matter how you feel your memory level is, do know that it can be improved on and sharpened to your desire. Not everyone's memory decline as they grow older, although the speed and accuracy of people begin to drop from their twenties, especially for those temporary memories containing information we use on a daily for decision making.

- **Lessons**
1. The last organ in the body to mature is the brain.
2. Our brain can process a visual image in a smaller amount of time than it takes for you to blink.
3. The hippocampus is the part of the brain known as the memory center.
4. The hippocampus is bigger in individuals whose jobs have high cognitive demands.
- **Issues surrounding the subject matter**
1. How is it that to remember, we have to learn to forget a bit?

_____
_____
_____
_____
_____

- **Goals**
1. Why is it that memory challenges are not predictable with age?

2. Explain the stages of memory building and how it applies to you?

- **Action steps**
1. In what ways can we continue to make the content of the memory to be constantly updated and changed but remain objective?

_____
_____
_____
_____
_____
_____
_____

- **Checklist**
1. Cognitive debility is not inescapable.

CHAPTER 2: COGNITIVE DECLINE—REDEFINED

Cognitive decline is often accelerated as an individual nears old age. For some, it is a fast decline process like a traumatic accident and for others, it is slow and steady. When the cognitive decline is in motion, we tend to wonder when it started, what may be the possible cause, what may be done to help the situation, not engaging in physical exercise, social activities, tasking jobs, and hobbies contribute to the acceleration of the disease, or eating disorders and even nutritional deficiency be the cause for cognitive decline?

Symptoms of cognitive decline are such as the following.
- Withdrawal from family and socializing.
- Puts a halt on personal hygiene.
- Becomes bad-mannered and utters offensive comments.
- Depressed and gives up on life and prefers to stir-away at the TV all day.
- Detaches from normal activities.
- Extreme forgetfulness.

Many factors are responsible for cognitive decline and its symptoms stream from long years of accumulated decline that has compiled and is now causing damage to the body. A young person at the age of fifteen can be on their way to Alzheimer's disease but have no idea. Even dementia isn't a subject to concern for many not until they clock fifty years old. Every young person should adopt a healthy lifestyle for them to keep waxing strong even in their old age. That walk to adopting a healthy lifestyle begins today.

The actual cause(s) of Alzheimer's disease is still not known with the advancement in medicine. This shows that humans are extremely complex beings. The reason for such difficulty and uncertainty in discovering the precise cause of the above disease is because what would cause lethal cognitive decline in Mr. A will not affect Mr. B, C, or D... The reasons behind the mind-boggling question above differ for everyone. Notwithstanding, there are some strategies and techniques we can adopt to reduce the possible risk of dementia.

What goes on in the brain of an Alzheimer's disease patient. As we know, the amyloid hypothesis explains that beta-amyloid are plagues of sticky protein that buildup in the brain and cause damage to the vital synapses that avails the brain cells to communicate effectively. Medications created to eliminate these plagues have failed in clinical trials time and time again.

The advancement of the disease is quite complex. Scholars keep investigating to know if the cognitive decline is the result of an increase in the normal aging process or it is caused by a degenerative disease of precise brain corridors. Possible triggers of the above disease as recent research shows are;

- Injury
- Persistent metabolic dysfunction
- Infection
- Nutrient deficiency
- Exposure to harmful chemicals

The above triggers encourage an immune reaction and inflammatory response that can damage the brain. Here are the most common causes of cognitive decline outside normal or enhanced aging. These are eight possible ways the brain starts to break as it reveals how lifestyle, genetics, and environmental factors add to the problem. The following outlined factors can be a large part of the problem than others, it all depends on personal risk factors.

EIGHT POSSIBLE WAYS THE BRAIN STARTS TO BREAK

1. **The Amyloid Cascade Hypothesis (ACH)**

Dr. Aloysius Alzheimer was the one to first give a detailed and documented report of symptoms describing the Alzheimer's disease which took his name to date. The deceased fifty-one-year-old woman experienced intense memory loss, displayed uncanny behavior, and perturbing/mysterious psychological changes.

His detailed report on the subject matter was available in 1907 after an autopsy was carried out on the disturbed late woman. The following was discovered in her brain;
- Dramatic shrinkage
- Abnormal deposits in and around nerve cells are called "senile plaques."
- The senile plaques contained beta-amyloid.

For over a century now, these amyloid plaques and neurofibrillary tangles stay as the trademarks of Alzheimer's disease. In the aforementioned disease, the amyloid plaques which gather among nerve cells and tangles entail tau protein which is twisted insoluble fibers inherent in the brain' cells.

Beta-amyloid and tau are essential in the brain. There are healthy versions to these proteins which are a healthy measure of the brain biology that helps to supply food to the cells of the brain and make sure vital chemicals move liberally among those cells. Trouble comes when the beta-amyloid and tau get damaged and turns into sticky clumps. When this occurs, the amyloid transforms into watertight rope-like structures carrying protein tightly fitted in. This interlocked formation sticks up to form dangerous plaques such as Alzheimer's disease.

The drugs responsible for reducing the functions of beta-amyloid in the brain is yet to be successful. A diseased brain doesn't show only one kind of damage inherent in the brain, there are a lot of damages present in an aging brain that can cause Alzheimer's disease. The complexity of this disease goes to show that there cannot be a universal solution due to the different dementias which calls for various treatments as well.

The human gene (genetics) can also be a factor. Mutation in the gene leading from genetic abnormalities sliding in for amyloid protein such as the amyloid precursor protein (APP) gene and presenilin 1 and presenilin 2 genes can be attributed for the early signs of Alzheimer's disease in individuals in families with this mutation due to the increase in beta-amyloid creation. In other families who have the genetic tendencies to grow early-onset Alzheimer's but end up being protected due to their other unique mutations, thereby showing no signs of cognitive decline even with neurological traces of the disease in question.

The issue of concern is the inefficiency and vulnerability of the body as it gets older to repair the system responsible for fixing DNA mutations. A typical example is the amyloid buildup described above because repair enzymes can't work anymore (just like in the case of cancer).

Neurofibrillary tangles (NFT) reveal a problem with tau protein. Tau proteins are responsible for soothing nerve cells in the brain and improve the level of communication in the brain. The occurrence of chemical changes in the brain means that the nerve cells can no longer hold it together; so they get knotted up and damaged.

Tau proteins are also associated with chronic traumatic encephalopathy (CTE) which is a progressive brain disease associated with recurring blows to the head and linked with depression, dementia, memory loss, and behavior problems. CTE is dominant in skilled athletes playing high-contact sports, such as football, boxing, soccer, and wrestling.

Blood Flow

Certain diseases affect the blood vessels. Plaques, and occasionally tangles are shown in individuals with high vascular disease. Thus, blood flow abnormalities in the brain may lead to Alzheimer's disease. Reduced blood flow to the brain leads to hypoperfusion which has been linked to the accumulation of plaques and tangles.

High blood pressure can result in infinitesimal destruction in the arteries principal to the brain, which can additionally reduce blood flow and oxygenation.

Metabolic Disorders

Here is another factor of concern bothering on dementia. Close to 85% of the U.S. population of adults are said to have metabolic syndrome, a mixture of health conditions such as insulin resistance, obesity, high blood pressure, poor lipid profile, and type 2 diabetes

In an autoimmune disease such as type 1 diabetes, there is resistance to insulin that should provide energy for the body because the cells responsible for such creation is destroyed. These folks settle for taking insulin shots since their bodies have a lot of the enabling grace to produce themselves. Studies have shown that individuals with high blood sugar at a greater risk of cognitive decline than individuals with regular blood sugar. APOE4 is the variant of the Alzheimer's gene and more evidence of this is found in type 3 diabetes.

Asides from the metabolic disorder for Alzheimer's disease; unhealthy weight gain has a part to play. There are cogent pieces of evidence that show that managing your weight can prevent brain decline later.

Toxic Substances

There are neurotoxins that we encounter that inflicts harm on us constantly, such as insecticides, pesticides, food additive, substances in plastics and harmful chemicals in our household good.

Other substances that can affect the functionality of the brain and be a potential cause of Alzheimer's disease are tetanus toxin (from bacteria), lead, and mercury.

Infections

As we have registered earlier that infections in the earlier part of life can lead the way for Alzheimer's disease decades later. Infections from different pathogens can lead to neurological effects. Scientists are now studying to see the forms of neurodegenerative decline and how the body reacts to these infections. Even mild infections affect the immune system in the brain and leave fragments tracks which births Alzheimer's.

DR. RUDY TANZI'S "ALZHEIMER'S IN A DISH"

Rudy Tanzi spearheaded the "Alzheimer's in a dish" in 2014 to understand Alzheimer's pathology. He and his team put mini-human brain organoids, clumps of brain cells used to develop "mini-brains", grew them in a petri dish, injected the Alzheimer's genes, and then watched what transpired. They followed and observed every interaction between the plaques and tangles and then what trailed; neuroinflammation and then noteworthy nerve cell death.

Dr. Rudy concluded his finding by saying that the "Amyloid plaques are the match, tangles are the brushfires, and neuroinflammation is the forest fire."

Other factors are; **Head Trauma and Injury, Immune System Challenges and Chronic Inflammation**

KINDS OF COGNITIVE DEFICITS

1. Normal aging
2. Mild Cognitive Impairment
3. Dementia
4. Normal versus not normal memory lapses (there are six types of normal memory lapses; **Absentmindedness, blocking scrambling, fading away, struggling for retrieval, Muddled multitasking**)

THERE ARE SEVERAL TYPES OF DEMENTIA.

- **Vascular Dementia -** caused by an impaired blood supply to the brain may be by a blocked or damaged blood vessel leading to strokes or bleeding in the brain.
- **Dementia with Lewy Bodies (DLB) -** This condition is very common among patients with dementia. Proteins, called alpha-synuclein or Lewy bodies build up in specific parts of the brain accountable for movement, cognition, and overall behavior. Consequently, patients have memory problems and indicators similar to Parkinson's.
- **Frontotemporal Lobar Dementia (FTLD).** Also known as Pick's disease, FTLD is a collection of disorders activated by gradual nerve cell damage in the brain's frontal and temporal lobes, causing changes in behavior.

- **Alzheimer's Disease.** This is a very common method of dementia. It is an advanced disease with symptoms that normally develop progressively before they intensify and become austere.
- **Lessons**
1. The buildup of plaques all over the brain cells is the main cause of Alzheimer's disease.
2. Cognitive decline is often accelerated as an individual nears old age.
3. Many factors are responsible for cognitive decline and its symptoms stream from long years of accumulated decline that has compiled and is now causing damage to the body.
- **Issues surrounding the subject matter**
1. What do you understand by cognitive decline?

_____
_____
_____
_____

2. Would you say the cognitive decline is normal or abnormal and why?

_____
_____
_____
_____

3. Is cognitive decline reversible?

_____
_____
_____
_____

- **Goals**
1. Would you agree that more research should be carried out to understand the chemicals that can result in brain abnormalities and why?

_____
_____
_____
_____

2. In your opinion, would you say that Alzheimer's diseases are over-diagnosed and why?

_____
_____
_____
_____

3. What do we need to do to prioritize the health of our brain?

_____
_____
_____
_____
_____

- **Action steps**
1. In what ways can we take care of our brain to increase its health, functionality and be able to build a new brain as we age?

_____
_____
_____
_____
_____

- **Checklist**
1. Focus on your brain and everything else will fall in place.

CHAPTER 3: 12 DESTRUCTIVE MYTHS AND THE 5 PILLARS THAT WILL BUILD YOU

The duty of a neurosurgeon requires living a life of purpose. The author explained how his journalistic skill and medical calling collide sometimes into a seamless rhythm. One time in 2003, he had to take off the journalist cap to put on his surgeon's cap to save a young lieutenant who had been shot in the back of the head in Iraq as he was the only neurosurgeon on site. This young man; Jesus Vidana survived the surgery in that uncertain setting and uncomfortable condition. The human brain is more resilient than you think. No matter how hurt the brain gets, it can be repaired under the right conditions.

THE DIRTY DOZEN

What does the human brain do and how does it change in the process of time? In trying to correctly answer the following questions and more, we need to first debunk the twelve most prevalent myths on the aging brain. This is just in a bid to help you know what can be done to de-age the brain and elongated its lifespan by introducing healthy habits. For this study, these myths are known as the "Dirty Dozen."

Myth #1: The Brain Remains a Complete Mystery

Everything is wrong about the above myth on all grounds. We have identified the various parts of the brain, their connections among different portions of the brain, and their level of relevance as it relates to our thoughts, feelings, and movement. Anatomically, we can identify the areas of our brain accountable for addiction, depression, and obsessive-compulsive disorder. The brain can be rejuvenated after injury or stroke.

Myth #2: Older People Are Doomed to Forget Things

There only lays a minute layer of truth in this myth. Some cognitive skills degenerate as we near old age, especially if we were too careless to make conscious efforts at helping ourselves remember when we tend to forget.

Myth #3: Dementia Is an Inevitable Consequence to Old Age

Dementia is not a standard part of aging. While the aging process can be slowed down for optimal health, diseases in old age can be avoided if the general bodily health is in top shape.

Myth #4: Older People Can't Learn New Things

The art of learning can take place at any given age; whether young or old especially when combined with cognitively stimulating undertakings like attempting new hobbies. The brain undergoes neurogenesis as it changes its capacity, information, and even learning strength. Even individual's diagnosed with cognitive decline and Alzheimer's disease can learn new things.

Myth #5: You Must Master One Language before Learning Another

Two languages and more can be learned concurrently because different parts of the brain don't go to war. There is no interference in any way, the brain can handle it.

Myth #6: A Person Who Has Memory Training Never Forgets

If memory training isn't enhanced each passing day, it will die.

Myth #7: We Use Only 10 Percent of Our Brains

This is a very old myth. It's ridiculous to be wasting away a whopping 90% of our brains; but does it stay ideal? If the above myth is anything to go by, then we all don't have anything to worry about as regards brain damage. The brain is like a town with houses, roads, and all linked up to make the town self-sufficient. Every component in the brain plays a major role there, no matter how minute.

Myth #8: Male and Female Brains Differ in Ways That Dictate Learning Abilities and Intelligence

Legend has it that women are better with issues bothering on intuition and empathy; while men are biologically suited for math and science. Biased research reveals that there are biological backings to the variances among both sexes. What is true is that the male and female brain is different in its functionality but none is better than the other, they are both unique. In America, it has been recorded that the number of patients with a higher risk of Alzheimer's disease is women; the reasons for this are still unknown.

Myth #9: A Crossword Puzzle a Day Can Keep the Brain Doctor Away

Word puzzles will not keep your brain young in the true sense of it. Although it is valuable to do Sudoku, word and number puzzles. What works is to constantly keep your mind active in other to reduce deterioration in thinking skills. If a crossword puzzle will do the trick; then do it.

Myth #10: You Are Dominated by Either Your "Right" or "Left" Brain

The two sides of our brains are convolutedly mutually supporting.

Myth #11: You Have Only Five Senses

Asides from the first five regular senses of the body are others that are equally processed in the brain and reveal a lot more about the body:

- Sight (ophthalmoception)
- Smell (olfacoception)
- Taste (gustaoception)
- Touch (tactioception)
- Hearing (audioception)
- Proprioception: It tells you where your body parts are and what they are doing.
- Equilibrioception: this is located in the inner ear giving you balance, also known as your internal GPS.
- Nociception: A sense of pain.
- Thermo(re)ception: A sense of temperature.
- Chronoception: A sense of the passage of time.
- Interoception: A sense of your basic internal needs, like thirst, hunger, needing to use the bathroom.

Myth #12: You're Born with All the Brain Cells You'll Ever Have, Your Brain Is Hardwired, and Brain Damage Is Always Permanent

HOW TO KEEP A SHARP MIND

How do we shape a better life? By building a sharper brain. These are the five pillars of brain health;

1. **Move** – Exercise is healthy for your brain (aerobics and nonaerobic). The movement tends to improve brain power by enhancing, repairing, and preserving brain cells in other to make them more productive and vibrant.
2. **Discover** – learning new things by the day is another way to keep your brain alive and strengthened.
3. **Relax** – Rest your brain when it needs to. Inefficient sleep can impair our memory and lead to chronic stress which can distort one's ability to learn anything new.
4. **Nourish** – a healthy diet is a must for a sharp mind. Foods like extra virgin olive oil, whole grains, cold-water fish, fibrous whole fruits and veggies, and nuts and seeds.
5. **Connect** – getting involved in various social networks can enhance the brain's plasticity and uphold our cognitive skills.

- **Lessons**
1. The five pillars of brain health are move, discovery, relax, connect and nourish.
- **Issues surrounding the subject matter**
1. How do we shape a better life?

_____
_____

2. What are your reservations about all the outlined twelve most prevalent myths on the aging brain?

_____
_____
_____
_____
_____
_____
_____
_____
_____

- **Goals**
1. Explain the ways to help in building a sharp mind?

_____
_____
_____
_____
_____
_____
_____
_____

2. In what ways can we successfully de-age the brain?

_____
_____
_____
_____
_____
_____
_____
_____
_____

- **Action steps**
1. What does the human brain do and how does it change in the process of time?

_____
_____
_____
_____
_____

- **Checklist**
1. If memory training isn't enhanced each passing day, it will die.

PART 2: THE BRAIN TRUST
HOW NOT TO LOSE YOUR MIND

The best antidote for illnesses, especially degenerative diseases that affect the brain and nervous system is prevention. Many adults today have no idea of the risk factors for dementia. How does one tackle a challenge they don't understand and see?

The strongest risk factor for Alzheimer's disease and dementia is "Age" and that isn't a subject matter that one can be taught to slow down; at least not yet. The aforementioned maladies occurrences are significantly higher as people approach sixty-five years of age and by eighty-five years old about a third of people would have been diagnosed with dementia as a result of compiling brain decline since when they were much younger.

Many people don't think about dementia when they are younger and do what it takes to prevent it from appearing as they advance in age. Asides from age as a risk factor for brain disease, there still exist other risk factors that can be controlled. That automatically tells us that we all have control over the risk of brain decline. The greatest modifiable and influential factors connected to brain decline and linked to lifestyles such as smoking, physical inactivity, social isolation, unhealthy diet, misuse of alcohol, lack of mentally stimulating activities, and poor sleep.

An average American has high blood pressure, is obese, has high cholesterol, diabetes which all increases the appearance of Alzheimer's disease and then dementia. The walk to prevention needs to start at an early stage. Here are tools that can help in preserving the health of your brain, its functions and it is all it the earlier stated pillars for preserving the brain's health and a twelve-week program to go with.

CHAPTER 4: THE MIRACLE OF MOVEMENT

Many don't know the miracle of physical movement in enhancing the brain's functionality and resilience to disease. A regular physical fitness routine is the grandest way to treat your brain. Don't relent or be downcast because you have never been consistent with working out in time past, today's decision can change that narrative and your brain and body will thank you.

Exercise is the only behavioral activity proven by science that triggers biological effects of great advantage to the brain. There aren't published documents that say that exercise will inverse cognitive deficits and dementia, but strong indications exist saying the rewards of getting in motion can reverse the above deficits and groom the entire body to function optimally. Starting today to get a better brain and body isn't impossible. Many people have achieved great feats and many more are still today such as; Ernestine Shepherd who began exercising at fifty-six years old, Madame Suzelle Poole at seventy-seven years old, Kazuyoshi Miura at fifty-some, Linda Ashmore at seventy-one, and John Starbrook at eighty-seven years old.

THE PACE OF AGING

In 2018, the American Academy of Neurology came up with fresh guidelines so that doctors infused exercise into patient's treatment to enhance the brain's functionality especially amongst those with a mild cognitive impairment which is an antecedent to dementia.

While there exist approved drugs by the FDA for the treatment of Alzheimer's dementia symptoms; there aren't FDA approved medicine for treating mild cognitive impairment (MCI). What scientists recommend is exercise. A study revealed that exercising at least two times weekly is beneficial to patients with cognition in MCI. Inactivity is the main demon we all are trying to tackle today, movement can help to heal the brain and give it the boost it needs to be renewed.

Amongst the authors of the new guidelines was a neurologist – Dr. Ron Petersen of "The Mayo Clinic". He is also a founding member of the Global Council on Brain Health. This world leader in the area of Alzheimer's disease research has given his life to studying cognition in normal aging, the various kinds of disorders like-

- Alzheimer's disease
- Lewy body dementia
- Frontotemporal lobar degeneration – this is a common form of dementia and it is a gradual loss of nerve cells in the frontal and or temporal lobes of the brain that leads to a decline in language, movement, or behavior.

Dr. Ron Petersen pressed on the benefits of exercise, most especially aerobics in preserving brain functionality. To date, physical activity still stands out in improving and preserving the overall functionality of the brain and the body as a whole. Choose the exercises that you want, if it is brisk walking, then start there. Regular physical activity is highly advised for not less than 150 minutes weekly. Incorporate interval and strength training alternatively to jolt the body's speed, effort, and intensity. This way the body will be able to withstand trying times. This mix of exercise will build muscle mass, tone the body, and brings about balance and coordination. Make out time from your busy schedule today, where there's a will, there is a way.

SMARTER AND BIGGER BRAINS IN MINUTES OF MOVEMENT

Exercise aids digestion, improves the body's metabolism, bone density, and body tone and strength. Exercise causes movements in the brain and can make us be smart genes, increase our self-worth and confidence asides improving our emotional stability, aiding weight loss, stave off depression and dementia. It is not magic, the reward of physical movement is seen and experienced when exercise becomes a lifestyle.

Exercise has ceased being just a form of leisure and sport, today it prevents illnesses and protects health. Inactivity causes the brain to shrink and increases the risk for Alzheimer's disease and other variances of dementia. Studies have revealed that being inactive no matter your body weight is worse than being obese. Prolonged sitting for more than eight hours a day without physical activity can lead to an individual's early death.

The damage is mostly metabolic. Immobility incites the accumulation of more sugar while the body isn't in circulation thereby suing less of your body blood sugar. Immobility negatively influences high-density lipoprotein (good cholesterol), blood fats, hormone leptin (it tells you when to stop eating), and resting blood pressure.

Prolonged sitting puts your muscle in a dormant state thereby diminishing the body's electrical activity, leading to degeneration and breakdown. At this point, the production of lipoprotein lipase is hindered leading to an increased amount of fat in circulation. It is simple; as your metabolic rate drops, you stop burning calories.

MOVING THROUGH EVOLUTION

Daniel E. Lieberman of Harvard; a Biologist and paleoanthropologist aware of the strength and benefits of physical activity on the physical frame and functions of the body.

The record has it that back in the 600 BCE—more than 2.5 millennia ago—Sushruta a physician during the Indus Valley civilization, was the foremost doctor to recommend judicious daily exercise for his patients and advised it should be done on a regular.

It is no longer news that for more than 2000 years ago, the medical community has recognized the link between the movement of the body and the health of the brain, and again it is beginning to take center stage.

BENEFITS OF EXERCISE
1. Lowers the risk of death from all causes.
2. Improves self-esteem and sense of safety.
3. Releases endorphins.
4. Decreases the risk for insulin resistance, diabetes, and blood sugar levels.
5. Aids an ideal weight circulation and maintenance.
6. Increases the health of the heart and aids lower risk for cardiovascular disease and high blood pressure.
7. Increases strength, energy, stamina, and flexibility.
8. Increases muscle tone and bone condition.
9. Increases oxygen supply to cells and tissues and blood and lymph flow.
10. Exercise aids better and sounder sleep.
11. It reduces stress.
12. It decreases inflammation and the risk for age-related disease, from cancer to dementia
13. It boosts the body's immune system.

SHAPE YOUR BRAIN BY GETTING INTO SHAPE

Exercising will not only get us into shape physically, but our brain will also get into shape. This is a given because exercise facilitates oxygenated blood flow, delivers nutrients for neural cell growth and preservation.

More so, exercise efficiently makes use of circulating blood sugar and decreases inflammation however motivating the release of growth factors that equally promotes the propagation and function of cells. These growth factors usher in new neurons, support their survival, and recruits blood vessels. The benefits of physical activity cannot be overemphasized, if the risk of high blood pressure, cognitive decline, Alzheimer's disease, dementia, and more illness can drastically reduce due to exercise, then we all have no defense.

JUST AS YOU WOULD BRUSH YOUR TEETH

Just as you will not negotiate to brush your teeth daily; so should exercising be for you. There are various kinds of exercises, a proper workout session is a combination of aerobic cardio workout such as cycling, jogging, swimming, strength training – weight lifting, lunges, gym machines, resistance bands, mat Pilates, squats, and for balance – yoga, stretches, etc.

Physical movement is a necessity for all, no matter your age; you can still be very much active. As you begin today, you will realize that you will begin to love it more and make it a lifestyle.

- **Lessons**
1. Exercising will not only get us into shape physically, but our brain will also get into shape.
2. Exercise aids digestion, improves the body's metabolism, bone density, and body tone and strength.
3. Exercise has ceased being just a form of leisure and sport, today it prevents illnesses and protects health.
- **Issues surrounding the subject matter**
1. How is the strongest risk factor for Alzheimer's disease and dementia "Age"?

_____

_____

_____

_____

- **Goals**
1. Based on the immense benefits of exercise on the general functionality of the body, how can this be indoctrinated into your lifestyle, draw out a worksheet if that will aid you better?

_____

_____

_____

_____

_____

_____

_____

_____

- **Action steps**
1. List out the types of exercise you have begun or will begin and what is your goal asides from attaining a sharper and healthier brain?

_____

_____

_____

_____

_____
_____
_____
_____
_____

- **Checklist**
1. A regular physical fitness routine is the grandest way to treat your brain.

CHAPTER 5: THE POWER OF PURPOSE, LEARNING, AND DISCOVERY

A study revealed that each extra year of work reduces the risk of getting dementia by 3.2 %. Staying longer and engaged in a job that gives you purpose keeps you physically active, mentally challenged, and socially connected all of which protect cognitive reasoning.

In Japan, retirement doesn't exist in their dictionary. During the author's search for the secrets of longevity, he learned from the Japanese in Okinawa, Japan. His stay in Okinawa, Japan taught him that delayed retirement is the way forward and even after retiring, we are not to quit on life. Still stay connected with your society, stay engaged, discover activities that bring your joy and warmth. Don't ever lose sight of your purpose even in a retired state. Continue to discover, learn and get the complex task completed. Every one of us' goal should be to age actively – this can only be possible when we have our sense of purpose intact, understand that our lives have meaning and direction and that there are still goals worth fulfilling.

KEEPING THE BRAIN PLASTIC

Active aging is more than physical exercise that involves recruiting the muscles for the overall wellbeing of the body. The one referred to involves challenging the brain in healthy ways in a bid to improve its health. Challenging the brain in the right way makes you unlock the rare attribute of the brain which is "plasticity." This helps the brain to rewire itself and fortify its connections.

During a brain autopsy, oftentimes patients don't act like the message their brain is tweeting. The information gotten from that autopsy stands contradictory to the owner's persona and can be very confusing. This brings to bother how possible is it that an individual with a sick brain escaped cognitive decline.

That can only be possible due to "cognitive reserve" or "brain resiliency" as tagged by scientists. Achieving the following has a lot to do with staying focused and engaged in meaningful things in life by participating in inspiring activities and socializing. Cognitive reserve is like a massive backup system inherent in the brain based on consequences from enriched life events such as occupation and education.

THE BRAIN AND COGNITIVE RESERVE

Cognitive reserve is a complex term that is hard to define. Cognitive reserve is the ability of the brain to improvise and find its way around challenges it may encounter in getting a job done. The brain's ability to always find alternative routes out of pressing challenges that could have harmed it and distort its functions is "cognitive reserve" or "brain resiliency."

The human brain should never be caught in a corner void of ways to turn around a bad situation/stuck position. Seeing the brain's networks as links of roads will help you understand that the more networks present; the more options there are to follow and still arrive at the same destination.

The roads or networks referred to here are the cognitive reserve which is developed by a long term of learning, through education, discovery, and curiosity. The stronger networks we build, the better it is for us to manage future disappointments or declines.

It's a simple way of looking at this, but those networks or roads are the cognitive reserves, and they develop over time through education, learning, and curiosity. The more you discover in your lifetime, the more networks you create to help your brain better manage any potential failures or declines it faces.

A group of scientists in the Department of Neurosciences at the University of California San Diego in the 1980s was the first to use the term "reserve" in their publication called "Annals of Neurology" when some advanced individuals in a skilled nursing facility with no outward symptoms of dementia had brains consistent with those of advanced Alzheimer's disease. The result was that these had enough brain cache to write off the impairment so they continued to function normally.

That discovery revealed that individuals who got away from symptoms of dementia have greater brain weights and much more neurons. People with a cognitive reserve can make insignificant the degenerative changes in the brain linked to dementia, other brain diseases like stroke, Parkinson's disease, or multiple sclerosis. The bigger your cognitive reserve, the more you can function better. Scientists advise that we expose ourselves more to brain triggers, unexpected life events that affect the brain like extreme stress, surgery, or toxins from our immediate environment. Anything that will joggle the brain extra such as learning, thinking, solving problems, and strategizing.

There are two types of cognitive reserve; neural reserve and neural compensation. Neural reserve allows established brain networks efficient enough to have a grander capacity less predisposed to disruption. Neural compensation allows alternate networks to counterpoise or balance out disruptions of previous networks.

An epidemiology report reveals that individuals with advanced education, higher IQ, occupational feats, or engaging in leisure accomplishments have reduced risk of developing Alzheimer's disease. So we can say it is a fact now that cognitive stimulation builds a brain that is resistant to diseases.

THE DEFINITION OF "COGNITIVELY STIMULATING" ACTIVITIES

Many people have the wrong understanding of cognitive stimulation. A lot of people go around saying that puzzle games and other brain games improve the health of the brain. Nine out of ten times, their position is just based on deception, no wonder the Federal Trade Commission has hampered down on companies tricking the public that their brain-training programs can be a protective covering against dementia and age-related cognitive decline.

While these games can improve the brain's ability to recall things and recover information; their advantages don't stimulate other brain functions like reasoning and solving problems. A secondary analysis funded by the National Institutes of Health of an original ten-year study in 2016 concluded that "speed training" was more operational than memory and reasoning exercises as it relates to potential effects on reducing the risk of developing dementia.

Dr. Gazzaley; the chief science advisor of Akili Interactive Lab that develops therapeutic games for treating brain disorders and a professor of neurology, physiology, and psychiatry at the University of California did his quota by making video games to help in treating brain disorders such as multiple sclerosis, attention deficit hyperactivity disorder (ADHD), autism, Parkinson's, Alzheimer's disease, and depression.

It is not enough to know the cognitive stimulating activities without purpose. Purpose only goes ahead to give you a drive and determination to make goals and see to it that they materialize. Don't stop climbing up the ladder, be optimistic enough to make your dreams come to light.

GETTING IN THE FLOW

This is a state of mind of being in the present. Don't just exist, live. Even if retired, enroll in classes to learn new things, teach if you love to, volunteer, horn your passion, work on your hobbies, renew your library card, be friendly with those around you and even your neighbors, do whatever makes life more joyful, meaningful, and satisfying. Living life aware of your present is living life in the flow, it shows you have a great purpose.

- **Lessons**
1. There are two types of cognitive reserve; neural reserve and neural compensation.
2. Active aging is more than physical exercise that involves recruiting the muscles for the overall wellbeing of the body. The one referred to involves challenging the brain in healthy ways in a bid to improve its health.
- **Issues surrounding the subject matter**
1. When last were you in the flow?
   _____
   _____

- **Goals**
1. What are cognitive stimulating activities and how does it apply to you?
   _____
   _____
   _____
   _____
   _____
   _____
   _____
   _____

2. What are the things to do to achieve active aging/brain plasticity?

_____
_____
_____
_____
_____
_____
_____
_____
_____

- **Action steps**
1. Write down the last experiences you had of when you were in the flow as these memories will aid you to find a new route to navigate the challenges of cognitive decline.

_____
_____
_____
_____
_____
_____
_____
_____

- **Checklist**
1. The bigger your cognitive reserve, the more you can function better.

CHAPTER 6: THE NEED FOR SLEEP AND RELAXATION

This a subject that many people struggle with, for some, sleep comes easy-peasy while for many others it is a tussle. Two-third of people in this time and age are consistently deprived of sleep. Sleep should make it to the top of everyone's priority list because of its immense benefits.

Many people say they can get by with little or no sleep just to get work done, but in the fact of it, they are putting themselves at risk of malignant health challenges.

Chronic sleep deprivation puts people at higher risk for the following;
- Depression
- Learning and memory problems
- Dementia
- Mood disorders
- Heart disease
- Weight gain
- High blood pressure
- Diabetes
- Obesity
- Cancer
- Fall-related injuries

Sleeplessness can also cause you to be behaviorally biased and make you unable to make wise decisions built on negativity. The body requires about seven to eight hours of sleep daily. Not sleeping isn't a badge of honor and tying your success to sleep deprivation is not the right way to go about the matter as you will get severely injured in the long run.

A professor of neuroscience and psychology at the University of California, Berkeley in the person of Dr. Matthew Walker is our generations' revolutionary researcher on the power of sleep. He mentioned that sleep is the third pillar of good health asides from diet and exercise. Recently he discovered that adequate sleep boosts the brain and nervous system, and can help in resetting our brains, bodies and increase life span.

Sleep isn't a useless and ideal phase. It is a time where the body replenishes itself in various ways that eventually affects our entire body system. Dreamless sleep and loud snoring are symptoms of sleep apnea (a sleep disorder) and waking up early is induced by the change in age, nevertheless, simple lifestyle changes can help to treat and improve sleep. Sleep apnea can be treated with the aid of continuous positive airway pressure (CPAP) device to be worn during sleep. People who are overweight get relief when they lose weight because the extra weight gained only impressed upon their airway causing fragmented sleep and regular interrupted breathing.

SLEEP MEDICINE

Sleep medicine has become rampant today to buttress the power of sleep to aid good health and mental wellness. Every creature on planet earth sleeps. Rats that spend most times of their lives awake die away in a month or days. Adequate sleep has amazing impacts on your overall well-being.

Adequate sleep keeps you alive, able to process information faster, sharp, attentive, and creative. Our sleep habits eventually rule over all that we are and what we are going to be, how large our appetite is, the rate of our metabolism, the strength of our immune system, your coping mechanism with stress, how insightful you can become, your inner strength at consolidating experiences in your brain and recalling things and how proficient you are at learning.

Various scientific backings reveal that a well-rested brain is a healthy brain free of "brain fog" and "brain shrinkage" due to high levels of inflammation. Sleep aids will help you fall asleep faster but they will not allow your sleep to be restful because it wasn't induced naturally. Some of these sleeping aids increase the risk for dementia, brain decline, insomnia, depression, anxiety, impairs thinking and balance.

THE RINSE CYCLE

Sleep has a way of washing/rinsing the brain off of toxic waste and fluid from tissues via the lymphatic system. This drainage passageway is now referred to as the glymphatic system. This fluid in the brain and spinal cord shields and bathes the central nervous system and removes waste products. Inadequate sleep hinders the brain from self-cleansing from debris, leading to extra amyloid that triggers Alzheimer's disease and more sleep deprivation.

THE TOP TEN SECRETS TO SLEEP
1. Stick to a schedule and avoid long naps.
2. Don't be a night owl.
3. Wake up to early morning light and absorb the sun.

4. Get moving, exercise regularly.
5. Watch what you eat and drink and the time you consume them too.
6. Mind your medicines.
7. Cool, quiet, and dark. Make the temperature ideal enough to aid quality sleep; between 60 and 67 degrees Fahrenheit.
8. Eliminate electronics. Keep your smartphones, TV screens, light bulbs, computer, and all away to help you concentrate and sleep.
9. Establish bedtime rituals. Engage yourself and your mind in activities that will calm your mind like about 30 mins before going to bed such as reading, a warm bath, drinking tea, listening to soothing music, or anything around that.
10. Know the warning signs. Watch your body and identify when sleep disorders kick in and their telltale signs.

Engage in relaxation exercises that help you meditate using yoga, progressive muscle relaxation, tai chi, guided imagery, breathing exercises, and repetitive prayer. Deep breathing is effective for triggering parasympathetic nerve responses and not sympathetic nerve responses that incite anxiety and stress. Deep breathing can be exercised anywhere to achieve lower blood pressure, a calm heartbeat, a deeply relaxed state, and slow breathing.

The below strategies can help you to become less depressed, anxious, socially isolated, and more resilient and brain-productive.

1. Find an additional hour in your day at least once a week for your "me time."
2. Establish a system of rewards.
3. Don't multitask—confront your day like a surgeon.
4. Recognize your marbles and sand in other to help you plan accordingly
5. Declutter your life. (Clean out your closets)
6. Become a regular volunteer in your community.
7. Express gratitude.
8. Exercise the art of forgiveness.
9. Look for things that make you happy.
10. Take breaks from email and social media.
11. Set aside fifteen minutes each day for yourself.
12. Allow yourself to daydream.
13. Do not be afraid to speak to a health professional if you have worries about your mental health.

Getting older is something honorable, it shouldn't be thought to trigger fear because we all will grow old one day, but how do we want to be when we are advanced in age? We all will say healthy and sound. But are we all doing what it takes now to make sure we are what we dream of? The journey to sound health begins today, don't live a life you would regret.

- **Lessons**
1. Deep breathing is effective for triggering parasympathetic nerve responses and not sympathetic nerve responses that incite anxiety and stress.

2. Adequate sleep keeps you alive, able to process information faster, sharp, attentive, and creative.
- **Issues surrounding the subject matter**
1. How do our sleep habits eventually rule over all that we are and what we are going to be?

_____
_____
_____
_____

- **Goals**
1. What are the activities you engage in that leave you less depressed, less anxious, less socially isolated, and more resilient and brain-productive?

_____
_____
_____
_____
_____
_____
_____
_____

2. In what ways will the rinse cycle benefit your overall wellbeing?

_____
_____
_____

_____
_____
_____
_____
_____
_____
_____
_____
_____
_____

- **Action steps**
1. Explain what sleep deprivation will cause you and what adequate sleep will bring your way.

_____
_____
_____
_____
_____
_____
_____
_____
_____
_____

- **Checklist**
1. Sleep is a compulsory segment of regeneration.

CHAPTER 7: FOOD FOR THOUGHT

Every year, the catalog of diet books and related materials keep compounding on various shelves and also on the internet. This increases the confusion on what is the right and ideal food our body needs whether it is for weight loss, to boost the brain's function, preventing heart disease, or more. There are various popular forms of diet ranging from vegan, Paleo, low fat, keto, pescatarian, gluten-free, low cholesterol, and low carb.

Even our health practitioners rarely give nutritional advice, most of the information people get is gotten from others and other undependable sources. With the aid of "data Dredging," we can see why there are so many contradictory headlines on nutrition. Today coffee, red wine, and cheese are seen to be protective against heart diseases, cancer, and dementia, and then the next minute, another literature comes to say otherwise.

So what is the best diet highly beneficial to the brain?
Certain lifestyle and nutrition go a long way to protect the brain and reduce the risk of major chronic diseases – cardiovascular disease, type 2 diabetes, cancer, and progressively dementia creeps in.

The ideal diet for your brain is an achievable way of eating with general guidelines and not a particular branded diet.
A cardiologist and nutrition researcher at Brigham and Women's Hospital in Boston–Sara Seidelmann, advised that eating every class of food in moderation is the way to go. She

said avoiding some classes of food is not a sustainable diet mode and can even lead to worse eating patterns later. We all are different, so getting a static diet for us all is impossible and unreasonable. Our metabolism rate differs and same as our food allergies. Focusing more on what you should eat rather than what you shouldn't make you end up eating foods rich in healthy calories than the bad ones. Asides from food being a source of nutrition, it should also be a source of enjoyment. Stop guilt-tripping yourself when you go out of your diet lane once in a while. Guilt is terrible for your brain and will only make you lose your sharpness and increase your cortisol and anxiety levels.

With a lot of complexities about the ideal diet that the brain needs, brought about the endorsement of the Mediterranean diet that was published in 2013 in the esteemed *New England Journal of Medicine.* This diet is rich in nuts, olive oil, fish, plant proteins, whole grains, wine with meals, vegetables, and fruits. This diet was found to be beneficial in lowering cardiovascular diseases, heart disease, and stroke, and individuals who followed the diet enjoy greater brain volume as they got older.

Late Dr. Martha Clare Morris, a professor of epidemiology at Rush University in Chicago, a founding member of the Global Council on Brain Health and director of the Rush Institute for Healthy Aging, discovered the MIND diet for a healthy brain aging, founded on centuries of findings into nutrition, aging and Alzheimer's disease. Acknowledging the limitations of nutritional studies, she was positive about the data-driven suggestions on the ideal food to be eaten that will positively affect the brain's health.

The MIND diet is a combination of the Mediterranean and DASH (Dietary Approaches to Stop Hypertension) modified to improve brain health. The "MIND diet" includes vegetables, beans, fish, nuts, whole grains, berries, wine, olive oil and stay clear of red meat, butter, cheese, pastries, and sweets.

WHAT'S GOOD FOR THE HEART IS GOOD FOR THE BRAIN

We need to be careful of food tagged "superfoods" said to help in protecting the brain such as juice tagged 100% fruits. Most of them are mostly sugar and void of what makes it pure and super. What is right for the heart is right for the brain – a heart-healthy diet is also a brain-healthy diet.

Dr. Isaacson developed new methods of cognitive testing in 2018. His work revealed that individuals can delay the progression of cognitive decline owing to the aging process may be by two or three years averagely by adopting simple lifestyle mediations and even if there was a preexisting family history of Alzheimer's disease. Patients are encouraged to work hand in hand with their doctors to not only improve cognitive functions but to reduce risk related to cardiovascular and Alzheimer's disease. This result encouraged people to take hold of their brain health.

Dr. Isaacson recommended some lifestyle strategies like sleep, exercise, and stress management. He advised that every patient should be given a personalized plan as no patient is the same even though there may be similarities in symptoms and pathology. Also Dr. Ornish of the Preventive Medicine Research Institute in San Francisco and his colleagues Dr. Bruce L. Miller, the director of the UCSF Memory and Aging Center played a vital role in dietary interventions to help treat and reverse, a wide collection of chronic diseases.

There is no single food that is said to be the key to good brain health but a combination of healthy foods can help to protect the brain from attack. Look for what works for you and add it to your routine to boost your productivity. Don't be afraid to start; it never too early or too late for you. Just start!

Drastically reduce your highly salty food intake, fast food meals, sugar and artificially-sweetened drinks, processed meats, and sweets.

MY GUIDE TO GOOD EATING

In an abridged version, here is a guide to healthy eating for the brain with the help of the acronym **S.H.A.R.P.**

S: Slash the Sugar and Stick to Your ABCs (sticking to your ABCs is to slash your sugar consumption and reduce your risk for dementia, insulin resistance, and blood sugar imbalances)

H: Hydrate Smartly (don't wait until you are thirsty to rehydrate, a lot of elderly people are rushed into the emergency rooms for dehydration. Try not to stuff yourself with food or by mistaking hunger for thirst. Dehydration can drain you of energy and your brain rhythm. Take note that alcohol is not a source of hydration even if it passes as part of a healthy diet)

A: Add More Omega-3 Fatty Acids from Dietary Sources (omega-3 fatty acids are gotten from nuts, seafood and seeds. It is brain-nourishing. Other sources of this fatty acid are mackerel, salmon, and sardines; plant-based source of omega-3 fatty acids canola, olive, soybean, flaxseed), nuts, and seeds (pumpkin seeds, chia seeds, and sunflower seeds)

Types of omega-3 fatty acids are ALA (alpha-linolenic acid), EPA (eicosapentaenoic acid), and DHA (docosahexaenoic acid) which is the most common of omega-3 fatty acid inside the brain which helps to maintain neuronal membranes.

R: Reduce Portions (eat your food in moderations/portions. Don't stay away from a certain class of food as our body needs all the nutrient it can get)

P: Plan Ahead (plan your meals so you are not caught eating junk food when hungry. Once you are hungry, your body craves for any available food in sight, don't destroy your long days of eating healthy because you failed to plan)

Other Tips

- Do Organic/Grass Fed foods.
- Spice things up using rich healthy spices like turmeric in meals. Always read the labels when grocery shopping.

The Gluten Debate

A gluten-free diet is a rampant phrase in this dispensation.

We now know that what is good for the heart is equally safe for the brain. Gluten has been linked to aiding risk in a heart attack. Only those who have been diagnosed with celiac can afford to go gluten-free and will reap tremendous benefits. Stay away from the gluten found in refined flours inherent in white bread, chips, crackers, and pastries. Get whole grain food that is great for your heart and brain health.

- **Lessons**
1. Supplements are only needed when your meals don't cover up for certain nutrients your body needs, so you take a supplement to augment it.
2. There are various popular forms of diet ranging from vegan, Paleo, low fat, keto, pescatarian, gluten-free, low cholesterol, and low carb.
3. Don't be deceived, there is no single food that is said to be the key to good brain health but a combination of healthy foods can help to protect the brain from attack.
4. Look for what works for you and add it to your routine to boost your productivity.
- **Issues surrounding the subject matter**
1. When should supplements and vitamins be infused into ones' lifestyle asides to make up for dietary imperfections?

_____
_____
_____
_____

2. What are your reservations about gluten-free foods?

_____
_____
_____
_____

- **Goals**
1. What are the ideal foods that are healthy for the brain and how do you intend to inculcate them into your life regularly?

_____
_____
_____
_____

2. Using the acronym S.H.A.R.P, shape your life. List out what you will infuse into your diet and what will be taken out.

_____
_____
_____
_____
_____
_____

- **Action steps**
1. What are the benefits of organic and grass-fed foods to the brain?

_____
_____
_____
_____
_____

- **Checklist**
1. Don't be afraid to start; it never too early or too late for you. Just start!

CHAPTER 8: CONNECTION FOR PROTECTION

The advantages of socializing outweigh its disadvantages – that is if there is any reason cogent enough to belong there in the first place. Being closely knitted with one's spouse impacts both their psychological perspective and physical health. The death of a loved one puts the other one at risk of mortality of about 41%. This is to buttress how the loss of a loved one puts the body at a higher risk.

A relationship of significance brings happiness, love, and security to a person's life. Asides from how meaningful relationship inspires psychological well-being, it is also linked to the outcome of our health – the endocrine, cardiovascular and the immune systems. Science has revealed that we need a social connection to flourish, especially in brain health. The results from the subject matter show that spending quality and purposeful time with the ones you love and contributing to meaningful social activities can help in keeping your mind sharp, strengthen your memory and improve your brain's functionality.

It was discovered by researchers at Michigan State University that married individuals are less likely to have dementia as they get older, but divorcees are just about twice as probable as married individuals to develop dementia. The widowed and yet-to-be-married stands in between the married and divorced group. With the high tendency that meaningful relationships can serve as a cushion against harmful effects of stress on the human brain.

Look around you, especially at the lives of elderly people who are still very sound and vibrant at a very old age. You will see the quality of their social network and their meaningful support system. Loneliness and social isolation are on the rise in our world today. It a silly paradox frenzy all over the world. We are hugely connected via digital media but yet still very much apart with loneliness oozing everywhere because of the void of authentic connection.

It is no longer news that the world lacks real connection and it has physical, emotional, and mental repercussions, especially for adults. This revelation has been buttressed by many expert bodies like- Global Council on Brain Health survey on socialization and the brain health of adults; Dr. Michelle C. Carlson, an issue expert for the Global Council on Brain Health, a professor at the Johns Hopkins Bloomberg School of Public Health in Baltimore, who partook in the review, called this challenge "a public health issue."

Specifically, loneliness has been revealed to increase cognitive decline in older adults. With all these said, this calls for maintaining and nurturing meaningful relationships in the same vein as you do your health through proper diet and exercise.

THE SECRET SAUCE TO A LONG, SHARP LIFE

How does connection affect our health? Harvard Study of Adult Development culled data recorded during the Great Depression in 1938 using the health of 268 Harvard sophomores. The result will be of great advantage to us all.

A psychiatrist at the Massachusetts General Hospital and a professor of psychiatry at Harvard Medical School in the person of Dr. Robert Waldinger is currently leading this study.

The doctor's findings exposed and debunked popularly believed myths about happiness and health.

Here are the lessons learned from Dr. Waldinger's research;
- Happiness and health are not about fame, wealth, or hard work.
- Happiness and health are about good and quality relationships.
- The quantity of your relationship doesn't matter, rather what matters is the quality of your relationship.

Note that our social networks can shrink as a result of retirement, death of a loved one, geographical separation, or an illness. Make extra efforts to find new connections to hinder the development of health and psychological challenges that may tend to arise as you grow older.

Close relationships with the ones you love will delay physical and mental decline, and shield you from life's displeasures, and guarantee you a happy and longer life span than any level of social class, wealth, fame, or IQ the world can offer. This is the truth, don't get it twisted.

TIPS TO HELP YOU STAY SOCIALLY ACTIVE
- Focus on the activities and relationships you enjoy the most; for example, an interest group.
- Make it a point of duty to reach out to your family, friends, relations, and neighbors regularly, whether physically or digitally.

- Maintain social connections with people of diverse ages.
- Volunteer at a school or community center.
- Search for programs around you that avail you of an opportunity to transfer your skills and knowledge to the next generation. Skills like; culinary skills, coaching a team, etc.
- Make it a point of duty to add new relationships or activities frequently. Position yourself in daily situations where you are sure to meet and network with others (e.g., stores or parks).
- Make efforts to have at least one reliable and trustworthy confidante to talk with consistently—somebody you can trust and count on.
- Anytime you feel isolated, speak to a professional, religious leader, or a therapist to help you understand what you feel.

The mere act of touching another human connects us with others to shield ourselves and them as well.

- **Lessons**
1. Quality relationships enhance the brain, and a healthy brain improves better relationships.
2. Being closely knitted with one's spouse impacts both their psychological perspective and physical health.
3. Asides from how meaningful relationship inspires psychological well-being, it is also linked to the outcome of our health – the endocrine, cardiovascular and the immune systems.
- **Issues surrounding the subject matter**

1. It is said that science reveals that we need a social connection to flourish, especially in the area of brain health; what happens when an individual tries all he/she can to make a solid relationship count and it still doesn't work. What other way can they get the benefits of a meaningful relationship based on the described scenario?

_____
_____
_____
_____
_____

- **Goals**
1. Mention all the ways you aim to begin to be socially engaged going forward?

_____
_____
_____
_____
_____

2. What is your understanding of—The quantity of your relationship doesn't matter, rather what matters is the quality of your relationship? And how do you intend to begin to make your relationships intentionally of quality?

_____
_____
_____
_____
_____

_____
_____
_____
_____

- **Action steps**
1. Draw out a timetable on the days and times you will spend quality time with those you love and contribute to meaningful social activities that can help in keeping your mind sharp, strengthen your memory, and improve your brain's functionality.

_____
_____
_____
_____
_____
_____
_____
_____
_____
_____
_____
_____
_____

- **Checklist**
1. It is no longer news that the world lacks real connection and it has physical, emotional, and mental repercussions, especially for adults

CHAPTER 9: PUTTING IT ALL TOGETHER
12 WEEKS TO *SHARPER*

Late Stephen William Hawking, a cosmologist, an English theoretical physicist, and author who was a director of research at the Centre for Theoretical Cosmology at the University of Cambridge helped the world see that every one of us "own" our brains, no one else does but you.

Every other thing can be taken away from you, but not your mind. That is exclusively yours and also the perception we have of the world.

What we see, smell, hear, taste, and touch goes through a lot of relay places, each altering the stimulus in ways that the ultimate version of the stimulus is greatly individualized. We all are distinct and unique beings, just the way no one else on earth carries your same fingerprint; let's aim to keep living our lives with that same uniqueness in mind.

No one said change is easy. It is stressful to alter long-standing habits to break into something entirely new. You will need to be strong-willed to make significant headway. And this time around, you need it to make healthy decisions that will benefit you now and even more in the long run.

THE BENEFITS THE "12 WEEKS TO SHARPER" WILL GIVE YOU
- Achieved less anxious thoughts.
- Better sleep.
- Enhanced energy.
- Less fogged mind.

- It puts you in a better mood.
- Makes you more resilient to regular stressors.

The five important goals you will achieve in these 12 weeks:

1. To be more active during the day and create an exercise routine into your life.
2. Discover novel ways to motivate your brain by learning and stimulating your mind.
3. Make your night rest a priority and integrate de-stressing activities into your daily routine.
4. Find new ways of nourishing your body.
5. Connect genuinely with others and keep a vibrant social life.

In the first week, you will begin five new habits daily based on the five pillars, and then repeat the new series of habits the subsequent week. During the third week, you'll integrate more habits into your days till you've gotten to the twelfth week with a whole new rhythm.

WEEKS 1 AND 2: DIVE INTO THE FIVE

Begin by addressing five areas in your life to work on for the next two weeks to get a better brain.

- **Move More** – inculcate an exercise you can practice regularly. Let your exercise be a mixture of cardio and aerobics; for not less than 30 minutes for at least five days in the week. Make sure to add strength training to your workout routine, at most three times a week; but give your muscle time to breathe and recover. Don't stick to exercise routines that keep you in your comfort zone, pull a surprise on your body, and use new muscles. A sedentary lifestyle kills us by the minute.

- **Love to Learn** – intentionally participate in cognitively stimulating activities. Learn new things, read books on different subject's asides from your profession of interest. Take up the challenge to learn a new language if you have always wanted to or any other skill.
- **Sleep Hygiene** – establish good sleep hygiene. Get about eight hours of sleep at night. If you never used to, work at increasing your sleep time. Some tips to help you achieve better sleep hygiene are – have your last meal of the day three hours before bedtime and stop caffeine at 2:00 pm, go to bed and wake up at about the same time, make your room conducive enough for resting and take out any form of distraction.
- **Eat Sanjay Style** – Eat only when the sun is up. Many have called this "Chrono" eating. When you eat is just as important as what you eat. Eat breakfast like a king, lunch like a prince, and dinner like a peasant. When you don't have time on your side and access to the kitchen, employ the **S.H.A.R.P.** method mentioned in chapter 7.

Some ideas for meal making:
1. Build a Better Breakfast – replace pastries with a proper meal such as – Steel-cut oatmeal with blueberries, cinnamon, crumpled raw walnuts, and a trickle of honey. There are healthier recipes in cookbooks. Instead of taking smoothies or juice, go for water, tea, or black coffee.

2. Smarter lunching – eat wholesome meals instead of fast foods. Switch your soda drinks for water, unsweetened tea, etc.
3. My Kind of Dinner – make your dinner making a lively session with family and friends, instead of grabbing fast-food. Also, try intermittent fasting if your doctor gives the go-ahead.
4. **Connect with People** – improve your social life and if you are already active; kudos to you.

WEEKS 3 AND 4

In your new routine, add at least two of the below;
- Call a neighbor over for dinner
- Embark on a twenty minutes' power walk after having lunch most days of the week.
- Add cold-water fish such as trout or salmon to your meal at least twice a week.
- Download a meditation app and begin to use it daily.
- Replace your soda drinks with water and tea.

WEEKS 5 AND 6

In your new routine, add at least three of the below;
- Make it a point of duty to own a gratitude journal. Every morning, spend at least five-minute writing down the people and things you are thankful for.
- Stay off processed foods.
- Add fifteen more minutes to your workout routine.
- Engage in relaxing activities before bedtime like mindful meditation.

- Attempt to go on a hike with friends or do yoga or Pilates.

WEEKS 7 AND 8

In your new routine, do the five ideas below;
- Visit your local farm to buy fresh foods.
- Make out time to volunteer in your community service.
- Book a checkup with your doctor and mention in detail your current medication and speak freely on your risk factors for cognitive degeneration.
- Try reading a subject or genre in an area of interest that you aren't used to.
- Write a letter to a younger loved one in your family, telling him/her an important thing you learned in your life and will love to pass over as a lesson, preferably handwritten.

WEEKS 9 AND 10

Ask yourself these questions and provide sincere responses.
- Are you getting thirty minutes of workout at least five times a week?
- Are you infusing resistance or strength training at least twice a week?
- Are you learning new things that can challenge my mind and develop various skills?
- Are you getting adequate sleep daily?
- Are you managing stress better?
- Are you adhering to the S.H.A.R.P. dietary protocol?
- Are you reaching out to family and friends regularly?

If the response to these questions is not in the affirmative, then you need to go through the sections that speak about them.

WEEK 11

This is the week to think about the ways you will want your family members to manage the news of a dementia diagnosis.

This is very sensitive to talk about, but it's best discussed with those you love.

WEEK 12

This is the week to list out all the things you did differently in the last several weeks and do a self-review to know if all your hard work worked, what didn't work and where can improvement come in. After tracing back to where you fell off, plan for a more productive week. Don't lose hope, progress is far better than perfection.

- **Lessons**
1. Every other thing can be taken away from you, but not your mind. That is exclusively yours and also the perception we have of the world.
2. We all are distinct and unique beings.
- **Issues surrounding the subject matter**
1. What are the possible barriers/hindrances that can come up to hinder your attaining the promising results for "twelve weeks to sharper?"

_____
_____
_____

- **Goals**
1. What are the things that you need to be done to get the result that you require?

2. Answer all the questions outlined above in weeks 9 and 10 in an orderly form.

3. List out all the things you did differently in the last several weeks and do a self-review to know if all your hard work worked, what didn't work and where can improvement come in.

   _____
   _____
   _____
   _____
   _____
   _____
   _____
   _____
   _____

- **Action steps**
1. What are the things/planning you think you need to put in place to get started with your first twelve weeks?

   _____
   _____
   _____
   _____
   _____
   _____
   _____
   _____

- **Checklist**
1. It is stressful to alter long-standing habits to break into something entirely new.

PART 3: THE DIAGNOSIS
WHAT TO DO, HOW TO THRIVE

The Marist Institute for Public Opinion carried out a survey that reveals that Alzheimer's diagnosis ignites fear in patients than other major life-threatening diseases such as stroke and cancer. The patient only starts to deteriorate when they have the diagnosis of dementia. Worse still, there are no drugs to cure it as there have been over four hundred failed attempts at drug trials costing billions of dollars. But, dementia isn't a death sentence even in the midst of these challenges. Dementia can be nipped in the bud; hope is not lost.

CHAPTER 10
DIAGNOSING AND TREATING AN AILING BRAIN

Instead of spreading fear and inordinate hope which is very unnecessary, we can channel our strength and drive to improvements in care and let the dementia patients and their caregivers know that it is a possibility to live optimally with the disease till a possible cure crops up.

Many people, even Bill Gates greatly fear losing his memory to dementia. In our search for the cure to dementia, scientists can alongside focus on coping strategies and early detection. This is very much important as finding the cure because amyloid gathers in the brain years before the symptoms show up and gives the patient a fighting chance to prevent the disease from becoming symptomatic even if not cured.

The idea of this book is not to pray that you won't have amyloid plaques in the brain, but that even though you do, it doesn't influence memory loss or other degenerating symptoms.

AARP which is a United States-based interest group that focuses on challenges affecting people over the age of fifty, United Health and Quest Diagnostics, and Bill Gates invested billions of Dollars in the discovery and development of revolutionary therapies for dementia in the Dementia Discovery Fund. To date, this research is still one with other bodies on board to fight this worthy battle to eliminate dementia.

BRINGING HOPE

It is a common practice for us to ignore symptoms and delay seeking medical help, but this is lethal. The Centers for Disease Control reported that only 13% of Americans walk in to report cases of experienced memory loss and confusion after age sixty while 81% are yet to reach out to a health care provider about their cognitive challenges. Alzheimer's doesn't just appear, it has been building up for many years and must have been leaving you tell-tale signs you blatantly ignored.

Notwithstanding, people can still live fulfilled and purposeful lives with a diagnosis of dementia. Giving up on life is not the best treatment for dementia, optimism and hope has a significant role to play in health and any diagnosis. Only those who hold on to hopefully get to live longer and fulfilled lives.

A POUND OF PREVENTION

The main tool for the treatment of dementia is prevention. What we need to do to reduce the risk of this malady is the same as what needs to be done to improve our quality of life with the disease. Dr. Richard Isaacson recounted that Alzheimer's disease begins in the brain for up to twenty to thirty years before its symptoms begin to show. Imagine if we are living healthy lives, exercising, eating right, socializing, and doing what we call a "Healthy Lifestyle" then the cells responsible for nurturing any trace of Alzheimer's disease will wither away as there is no fertile foundation to grow it. The above disease, cognitive decline, and dementia can be retracted if we do what we are supposed to at the early stage of our lives.

WHEN SHOULD I GET TESTED FOR THE ALZHEIMER'S GENES?

Get tested under close observation of a physician to discover if you have the Alzheimer's gene. Most importantly, your lifestyle habits affect your brain more than would any gene.

THE THREE STAGES OF ALZHEIMER'S DISEASE

- Mild (early stage),
- Moderate (middle-stage), and
- Severe (late-stage).

The stages differ in their projection and it affects the symptoms' speed and severity. Depending on the stage of the disease, it can be said to be benign or malignant.

The Alzheimer's Association reviewed the above stages below;
- **Early Stage: Mild Alzheimer's Disease**

Here, an individual still functions self-sufficiently and socializes just fine. Until an unusual memory decline strikes. They begin to face difficulties like; finding it hard to recall names of newly introduced people, struggling to find the appropriate words, fighting to perform work task, finding it hard to recall recently read materials, misplacing valuables, difficulty in planning and organizing, mood, and personality swings, social withdrawal, altered vision and struggle to communicate.

- **Middle Stage: Moderate Alzheimer's Disease**

This stage lingers for many years. As the disease develops and the symptoms become greater; those diagnosed with Alzheimer's disease will require better care as they begin to struggle to carry out their formally normal daily routine. Its symptoms are; frustration, confused thoughts, being erratic, forgetting important dates significant to them, moody feeling, withdrawal, forgetting personal contact details, struggle with controlling bowel and bladder, distorted sleep pattern, wandering lost, highly suspicious and delusional, repetitive behavior over and over.

- **Late Stage: Severe Alzheimer's Disease**

At this stage, their cognitive ability is far declined. They struggle to communicate efficiently, have control over their movement, or respond to their environment. It becomes difficult to express their feelings of pain, joy, etc.

The test to help detect Alzheimer's disease doesn't search out the subject matter, it instead reveals other causes of the patient's symptoms like small or large strokes, tumors, a buildup of fluid in the brain, or damage from severe head trauma. Structural imaging with magnetic resonance imaging (MRI), computed tomography (CT), and PET are the ideal medical checkups for Alzheimer's disease.

DEMENTIA IMITATORS

- Normal Pressure Hydrocephalus (NPH) – this is a gradual accumulation of cerebrospinal fluid (CSF) inside the brain, resulting in swelling and pressure that can destroy brain tissue in the long run.
- Medications – everyone has gone on a frenzy of prescription drugs without stopping to think of the side effects. They take Antibiotics, antidepressants, benzodiazepines (for sleep and anxiety), opioids, statins, and blood pressure medications. We throw caution into the wind and create dementia imitators with the intake of drugs.
- Depression – serious depression can cause symptoms of dementia called "pseudodementia." If a person's depression is cured, it improves their cognitive impairment. But that individual still stands a chance of still being brought down by dementia later.
- Urinary Tract Infection (UTI) – this is a result of an accumulation of harmful bacteria in the bladder, kidney, urethra, and ureters. In older persons, the symptom is like that of dementia. Treating the infection properly can help to ease the symptoms felt.
- Vascular Dementia – this is caused by various numbers of adverse cardiovascular conditions involving a

massive stroke where functions are lost in some parts of the body (mini-strokes) or struggle with speaking.
- Nutritional Deficiencies - The Global Council on Brain Health's report on supplements advised that using supplements for brain health is not advisable unless a health care provider has instructed you to do so for a nutritional deficiency.
- Underlying Infection – Some infections can activate symptoms of dementia.
- Brain Tumor – benign brain tumors may not pose any threat and even if they do, they can be surgically removed not like the plaques causing Alzheimer's dementia.
- Subdural Hematoma from a Head Injury
- Alcohol Misuse (alcohol dementia)

THE MEDICAL CHECKUP

A dementia medical workup should include these;

- Take note of current and past maladies.
- The patient's medical history and total physical and lab work.
- History of Cognitive and behavioral alterations and psychiatric history.
- Past and current illnesses.
- Medications and supplements taken
- Any medical condition affecting other family members.
- Lifestyle habits like exercise, diet, and intake of alcohol.

Types of tests to identify potential problems:

- The Alzheimer's Disease Assessment Scale–Cognitive Subscale (ADAS-Cog)
- The Mini-Mental State Exam
- The Mini-Cog test
- The Self-Administered Gerocognitive Examination (SAGE

SOME OF THE NATIONWIDE ORGANIZATIONS/PROGRAMS LOOKING INTO DEMENTIA:

- AARP
- The Cleveland Clinic's Lou Ruvo Center for Brain Health
- The Dementia Action Alliance
- The Family Caregiver Alliance
- The Mayo Clinic's Alzheimer's Disease Research Center
- The Memory Disorders Program at New York-Presbyterian/Weill Cornell Medical Center
- The National Institute on Aging funds Alzheimer's Disease Research Centers (ADRCs)
- UCLA's Alzheimer's and Dementia Care Program

TREATMENTS: DRUG-BASED AND PEOPLE-BASED

These two kinds of drugs often are prescribed together, particularly in later periods of the disease. The two FDA-approved classes of drugs to reduce symptoms of Alzheimer's disease aims to keep brain cells connecting but these therapies are not so promising and come with their side effects.

1. Acetylcholine –contains cholinesterase inhibitors.
2. Memantine (Namenda).

- **Lessons**

1. No single diagnostic test can determine if a person has Alzheimer's disease.

2. In dementia, the caregiver is more important than the doctor.
- **Issues surrounding the subject matter**
1. Why do many fear losing their memory to dementia?

_____
_____
_____
_____
_____

- **Goals**
1. When would you say is the ideal time to get tested for Alzheimer's genes and why?

_____
_____
_____
_____

- **Action steps**
1. What should a standard dementia medical workup include, list them out?

_____
_____
_____
_____
_____
_____
_____

- **Checklist**
1. No one is ever prepared for dementia, live while you can.

CHAPTER 11: NAVIGATING THE PATH FORWARD FINANCIALLY AND EMOTIONALLY, WITH A SPECIAL NOTE TO CAREGIVERS

The job of caregivers to one diagnosed with dementia isn't easy. This time is often a challenging period for the family and depending on their former bond, this diagnosis can either make them stronger or break them finally. Some family members cannot handle the stress that comes with caring for a cognitively impaired patient and whisk them off to a health-care facility to care for them, they won't mind the exorbitant cost.

Some of these facilities advertised as specializing in memory care are unsafe for these patients, the food goes bad and is still served to them, the care is nothing to write home about, and some of the patients are abused and mistreated. Even with this insight, more memory care living facilities are still being built and is now the fastest-growing sector of senior care.

IT TAKES A VILLAGE

A model village called De Hogeweyk lay within the city of Weesp, few minutes outside the Netherlands' capital city of Amsterdam. This was a definition of distinction in the way patients with advanced dementia were treated and made to live out for the rest of their lives. This facility was founded by two Dutch women who worked in traditional extended care facilities and decided to build a conducive home where their parents with progressive dementia can live their best lives even with their recent diagnosis. This notion guided them to build "De Hogeweyk."

De Hogeweyk is tagged "Dementia Village" of twenty-three two-story dormitory-style with the intricacies that replicates the real world, see them below;
- Guards guide the single pair of sliding glass doors that separates Hogeweyk from the outside world.
- There is only one way in, one way out.
- The surrounding was an embroidery of Dutch tulips wrapped around bubbling fountains.
- Made up just to look like an attractive Midwestern college campus with its combo of dormitories, streets, cafes, squares, restaurants, bar, salon, theaters, and street musicians.

Hogeweyk designed everything to meet the needs of those who suffer a cognitive decline as they advance in age. Those from the upper-class group had their place designed to touch and attend classical concerts, just so they are not missing home for any reason, and were the others. They were grouped according to their skills, disciplines, and interest so they are around those who will leave a significant impact on their lives.

A place of worship is available for religious people, they are made to manage themselves, cook and wash with the help of a caregiver. A currency was used in exchange for groceries as patients walk to the market to buy what they want – although that currency only circulated inside the village. They are encouraged to gather outside in the gardens or other recreational centers so they are not inside all day. There aren't nurses in white lab coats and all the theatrics that is accustomed to the conventional dementia care system. These attributes and more makes De Hogeweyk specialized in eldercare.

After some time, occupants of Hogeweyk became more joyful, took less sedating medications, had an improved appetite, and lived longer than those in customary elder care facilities. Hogeweyk is popular for their painstaking care and attention to their residents till they die happily. The Dutch government subsidizes the health care bills for dementia patients to residents depending on their income and it never exceeds $3,600. This is still operational to date.

The Hogeweyk experience revealed the various ways dementia touches the brain to keep it engaged. Lessons "Dementia Village" taught the author;

- Fight the urge to correct a dementia patient.
- Don't force them to retrieve an experience they no longer recall in their brain.

BRACE YOURSELF

Most of the caregivers of dementia are middle-aged females, an older female child, or the partner of the one down with dementia. Approximately 75% of individuals in the U.S. suffering from dementia are been taken care of by close family members and friends (mostly females). This is not a time to cry and let depression get the better part of you, you have to take care of these loved ones who would have taken care of you if the case was reversed. Brace yourself in ways that even after the journey is over, you haven't lost yourself to the battle.

These caregivers get so lost and immersed in offering care to Alzheimer's disease patients that they forget to cater for their health and may come down with the same disease. In America, the most caregivers for Alzheimer's disease are women, almost two-thirds of Americans with the disease are women, with the female estimated lifetime risk of developing Alzheimer's disease at sixty-five years of age is 1 in 6; in comparison to 1 in 11 women for breast cancer.

Recently, reports have revealed that other factors make the female folk more prone to the above disease such as;

- Due to biological disparities owing to perimenopause, scholars pay close attention to the protective/destructive effects of progesterone and estrogen.
- Symptoms of tau protein are already significantly spread in a woman's brain that is in the early phases of Alzheimer's disease compared to men.

When many families will love to outsource the care of their family members diagnosed with Alzheimer's to a caregiver, they run away from it because it is very expensive. And that won't change anytime soon due to the steady increase in cognitive decline diseases.

See more useful information on Alzheimer's disease on the following free platforms;
- Alzheimer's Association
- AARP
- Global Council on Brain Health

STEPS TO TAKE IMMEDIATELY AFTER A DIAGNOSIS
- Where to find support and education programs in your local area.
- Where to find early-stage social engagement programs.
- Where to find clinical trials same needs.
- Ways to keep a home safe.
- Ways to make a legal plan.
- Ways to make a financial plan.
- Ways to build a care team.

KEEP TALKING

Keep an open conversation with your family earlier to avoid a court-appointed conservator immediately after your Alzheimer's diagnosis is confirmed. Call extended family members to gather in this meeting for moral support. For those that cannot make it to the meeting, use applications that can make them virtually present. The idea is that everyone has firsthand information on the new development. Have your trust prepared as soon as possible, preferably when you are done with this reading. This an emotional subject matter to talk about but it is essential.

DON'T FORGET YOURSELF: A NOTE FOR CAREGIVERS

Caring for a loved one with dementia shouldn't be left to just a member of the family because that is very draining. It requires a team effort of friends and family members. The primary caregiver is the main point of contact responsible for the patient while the others do a good job at supporting. Thus, this primary caregiver must prioritize self-care while taking care of the patient.

Here are some of the things a primary caregiver should do;
- Be diligent with a healthy diet
- Exercise regularly
- Do activities that stimulate your well-being
- Spend quality time with your family and friends.
- Take out time to rest well from your caregiving duties
- Have a to-do-list of your own, don't live your entire life catering for a sick person, it is psychologically draining.
- Put a check on your emotions, manage your time and energy well.

Caregivers tend to burnout due to the rigorous responsibility of their duties but more because they neglect their physical, emotional, and spiritual health. When the job becomes a lot to handle, don't be embarrassed to get help for yourself and the one you love.

As a family caregiver, find your motivation (love, duty, or guilt) to help ginger you as you take care of the patient. It will serve as a constant reminder in challenging times.

Family Caregivers face guilt and denial at the onset of their duties. They can't just understand why a loved one will suffer at the hands of a cruel disease like Alzheimer's. No one is prepared for most of the things life throws our way, but we step forwards into the battle ring and fight for our survival and that of those we love.

The caregiver's goal is to care for the dementia patient at all costs. This isn't an easy job and it may come with little or no gratitude, so brace up and pat yourself at the back. You are doing what most people can't do and will never do.

- **Lessons**
1. Family Caregivers face guilt and denial at the onset of their duties.
2. Caregivers tend to burnout due to the rigorous responsibility of their duties but more because they neglect their physical, emotional, and spiritual health.
3. Most of the caregivers of dementia are middle-aged females, an older female child, or the partner of the one down with dementia.
- **Issues surrounding the subject matter**
1. What should an individual who has just been diagnosed with a cognitive decline disease do immediately it is affirmative?

_____
_____
_____
_____
_____

- **Goals**
1. Do you think that De Hogeweyk's experience will work in the United States and why is your response so?

_____
_____
_____
_____

_____
_____
_____
_____
_____
_____

2. List out all the lessons you learned from the De Hogeweyk facility and how it can be infused into the American Health Care System.

_____
_____
_____
_____
_____

3. As a caregiver, what are the things you need to know to carry out your duty efficiently?

_____
_____
_____
_____
_____
_____
_____
_____

- **Action steps**
1. As a caregiver document your journey in a summary here.

_____
_____
_____

_____
_____
_____
_____

- **Checklist**

1. The duty of a caregiver isn't a walk in the park, it requires a lot of patience, dedication, and commitment.

CONCLUSION
THE BRIGHT FUTURE

The world will not stop in its drive to find better treatments for Alzheimer's or even a possible cure. Research has been conducted looking for a possible solution but still no headway. The same happened in 2019 when a vaccine hit the scenes at the University of New Mexico by some scientists. The experiment was targeted at tau protein reduction and the mice were injected with tau protein as the objects of this experiment. The mice grew antibodies that eliminated the injected substance from the aspect of their brain associated with memory and learning. But can this work on humans and reduce dementia effects? It is yet to be proven.

A different team of scientists is working on "endobody" vaccines to boost the immune system to tackle malfunctioning internal parts of the body that we will overlook on a normal day. More clinical trials are ongoing to see that this vaccine will have a positive impact on memory and cognition which will take several years for results to come in. Notwithstanding, researchers are still working round the clock to make sure there is an end to the kinds of diseases linked to the brain like mental disorder, bipolar disorder, and neurodegenerative diseases.

With all of the above in mind and more, let's get to work. If we need to change our habits, now is the time to. Living your best life starts now, how do you want to be remembered? Begin to shape that thought in the minds of those you love today.

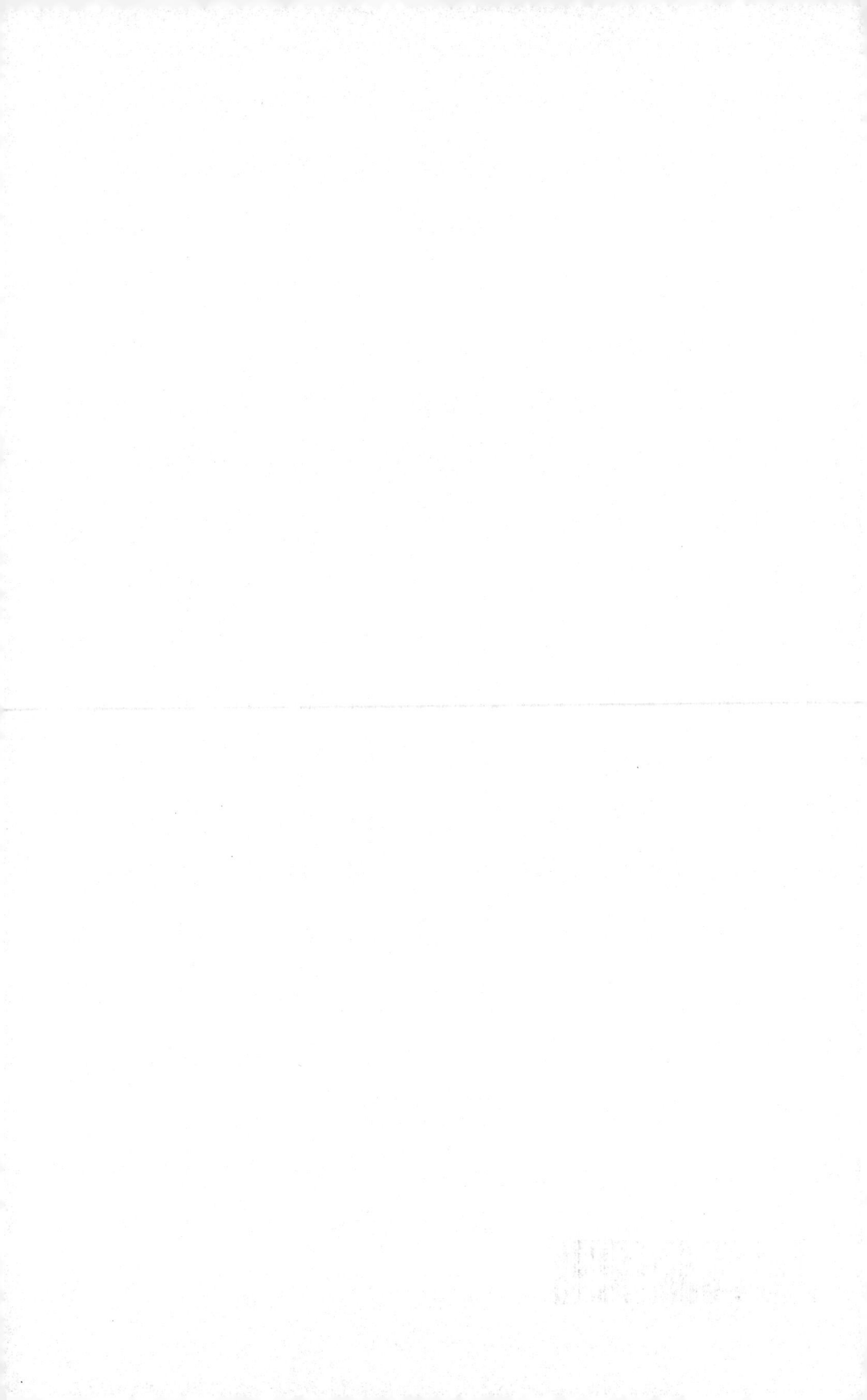

Made in the USA
Middletown, DE
05 May 2021